Contents

C000193655

Serum biochemistry

Biochemistry	Normal values	Significance	Deficiency	Excess
Potassium (K⁺)	3.5–5 mmol/l	Major intracellular cation Necessary for the generation of a nervous impulse and muscle contraction	Muscle weakness and fatigue Cramps or paralysis of the bowel leading to constipation Dizziness, confusion, arrhythmias	Muscle cramps Arrhythmias leading to cardiac arrest
Sodium (Na⁺)	135–145 mmol/l	Major extracellular cation Important for water balance in the body Necessary for the generation of a nervous impulse and contraction of muscle	Muscle weakness and lethargy Muscle cramps Dizziness High blood pressure and oedema Fits or coma	Postural hypotension leading to confusion Oliguria (if water deficient) Thirst Dehydration leading to dry, flushed skin Fits or coma
Calcium (Ca⁺)	2.1–2.65 mmol/l	Important for nervous impulse generation and muscle contraction Maintenance of bones and teeth Blood coagulation	Tetany (laryngeal spasm/stridor) Muscle spasm due to increased nerve excitability Low blood pressure Renal failure	Imbalance of muscle activity Muscle weakness and lethargy Muscle atrophy and weight loss High blood pressure Polyuria, polydipsia Depression
Albumen	35–50 g/l	Important for generating osmotic pressure	Oedema, oliguria Low blood pressure	Dehydration, polyuria High blood pressure
Glucose	3.5–5.5 mmol/l (fasting)	Vital for cellular respiration	Hypoglycaemia leading to: hunger, sweating, tremor, drowsiness, personality change, fits or loss of consciousness	Hyperglycaemia leading to: polyuria, polydipsia, lethargy, ketonic breath, anorexia, dehydration, vomiting, coma

Blood gases and useful biochemistry

BLOOD GASES

Biochemistry	Normal values	Significance	Deficits/excess	
Oxygen (PaO$_2$)	11.3–14 kPa	Vital for cellular respiration	Hypoxia (reduced arterial PaO$_2$): Cyanosis of tissues observed in tongue, mucous membranes (eye) and skin Increased respiratory rate Restlessness, confusion Acidosis (pH below 7.36) leading to cardiopulmonary arrest	
Carbon dioxide (PaCO$_2$)	4.6–5.6 kPa	Waste product of cellular respiration	Excessive loss of CO$_2$ leading to alkalosis (pH above 7.44)	Retention of CO$_2$ leading to acidosis (pH below 7.36)

OTHER SELECTED BIOCHEMISTRY

Biochemistry	Normal values	Significance
Sulphate Phosphate Urea Uric acid Creatinine	83–125 micromol/l 0.9–1.3 mmol/l 2.5–6.7 mmol/l 0.18–0.42 mmol/l 70–150 micromol/l	Nitrogenous wastes which are the breakdown products of cellular metabolism Excessive levels lead to acidosis (pH below 7.36)
Chloride	95–103 mmol/l	Anion important for maintaining fluid balance through osmotic pressure
Iron	13–32 micromol/l	Component of haemoglobin molecule A deficiency of iron will lead to anaemia causing tiredness and pallor
Cholesterol	4–<6 mmol/l desired	Important dietary lipid Constituent of cell membranes

Coagulation tests:

Prothrombin Time (PT) – time taken for clotting of citrated plasma after the addition of calcium and standardized reference thromboplastin, and expressed as the ratio of the PT of the patient to the PT of a pool of plasma taken from healthy subjects on no medication.
Activated Partial Thromboplastin Time (APTT) – common laboratory technique used with heparin treatment.
International Normalised Ratio (INR) – the internationally recommended form of reporting prothrombin time when measuring warfarin.

Urine chemistry

Definition: urinalysis is the testing of the physical characteristics and composition of a fresh specimen of urine. Urinalysis is a test that assists in establishing a preliminary diagnosis and identifies the need for further investigation. Urine forms in the kidneys, which process approximately 180 litres of blood-derived fluid a day. Roughly 1.5% of this total actually leaves the body. Fresh urine usually has a slightly aromatic odour; this can alter as a result of disease processes, e.g. diabetes mellitus when acetone is present and a slightly fruity smell occurs.

Urine chemistry: urine electrolytes reflect the ability of the kidney to excrete and reabsorb electrolytes

Sodium	100–260 mEq/24 hours
Potassium	39–90 mg/24 hours
Calcium	100–300 mg/24 hours

Abnormal results may be caused by a range of disease processes other than renal disorders, e.g. raised calcium, due to prolonged immobility.

Test	Normal	Abnormal
Colour	Amber-yellow	Red indicates haematuria (possibly urinary obstruction, renal calculi, tumour, renal failure, cystitis)
Clarity	Clear	Cloudy: debris, bacterial sediment (urinary tract infection, UTI)
pH	4.6–8.0 (average 6.0)	Alkaline on standing or with UTI; increased acidity with renal tubular acidosis
Specific gravity	1.003–1.030	<1.025 on random urine test
Protein	0.8 mg/dl	Proteinuria may occur with high protein diet and exercise (prolonged); seen in renal disease
Sugar	0	Glycosuria occurs after a high intake of sugar or with diabetes mellitus
Ketones	0	Ketonuria occurs with starvation and diabetic ketoacidosis
RBCs	0–4	Injury to kidney tissue (refer to colour, above)
WBCs	0–5	UTI
Casts	0	UTI, renal disease

Sources/bibliography: 1. Mallett J, Dougherty L. (eds) (2000) *Manual of Clinical Nursing Procedures.* Royal Marsden Hospital. Oxford: Blackwell Science. 2. Marieb E. (1998) *Human Anatomy and Physiology,* 4th edn. California: Benjamin Cummings. 3. Phipps W, Cassmeyer V, Sands J, Lehman M. (1995) *Medical Surgical Nursing. Concepts and Clinical Practice,* 5th edn. St Louis, Missouri: Mosby.

Blood composition and measurement

Component	Volume	Normal values
Blood cells	Make up 45% of blood volume	Cell counts: Erythrocytes: male $\quad$ 4.6–6.2×10^{12} per l female $\quad$ 4.2–5.4×10^{12} per l Leucocytes $\quad$ 4.5–11×10^{9} per l Platelets $\quad$ 150–400×10^{9} per l Haematocrit: male $\quad$ 0.4–0.5 mmol/l female $\quad$ 0.37–0.47 mmol/l Haemoglobin: male $\quad$ 2.17–2.79 mmol/l $\quad\quad$ (13–18 g/dl) female $\quad$ 1.86–2.48 mmol/l $\quad\quad$ (12–16 g/dl)
Plasma	Makes up 55% of blood volume	Plasma (90% water): albumin 35–55 g/l, globulin, fibrinogen, clotting factors, inorganic salts, nutrients, organic wastes, hormones, antibodies, gases

Sources/bibliography: 1. O'Tool M, Keane CB. (1997) *Encyclopedia and Dictionary of Medicine, Nursing and Allied Health*, 6th edn. Philadelphia: WB Saunders. 2. Watson R. (2000) *Anatomy and Physiology for Nurses*, 11th edn. London: Harcourt Publishers. 3. Ross J, Wilson JW. (1990) *Anatomy and Physiology in Health and Illness*, 7th edn. London: Churchill Livingstone. 4. Hoffbrand AV, Pettit JE. (1994) *Essential Haematology*, 3rd edn. Oxford: Blackwell Science. 5. Longmore M, *et al.* (2001) *Oxford Handbook of Clinical Medicine*, 5th edn. Oxford: Oxford University Press. 6. Tortora GJ, Anagnostakos NP. (1987) *Principles of Anatomy and Physiology*, 5th edn. London: Harper & Row. 6. Alexander MF, *et al.* (1999) *Nursing Practice: Hospital and Home, the Adult*, 3rd edn. London: Churchill Livingstone.

Cellular composition

Blood cells	Products for infusion	Uses	Description	Cell types		Characteristics and function
Red blood cells (erythrocytes)	Whole blood	Loss through trauma or surgery	Reduced platelet and clotting factors Freezing increases shelf life Washing removes surface antigen			No nucleus, contains haemoglobin Main function is the transport of oxygen to cells and carbon dioxide away from cells Produced in the bone marrow
	Packed cells, frozen red cells, washed red cells	] reduced cells				
White blood cells (leucocytes)	White cell concentrates	Acute leukaemia Aplastic anaemia Neutropenia	Not used very often Important to do tissue typing to prevent incompatibilities Steroids and antihistamines may be given	Polymorpho- nuclear leucocyte		Neutrophils (40–75% of white blood cells): ingest bacteria and debris Eosinophils (1–6%): protect body against foreign materials Basophils (0–1%): contain heparin and histamine necessary for vasodilation
				Lymphocyte (20–45% of white cells)		Important in the production of antibodies
				Monocyte (2–10%)		Performs phagocytotic activity
Platelets (thrombocytes)	Platelets	Patients suffering from thrombo-cytopenia due to aplastic anaemia; patients on myelotoxic chemotherapy	The platelets used for infusion are collated from many different blood units therefore steroids and antihistamines may be used			No nucleus Disc shaped Necessary for the clotting of blood

Blood groups

Blood grouping is determined by two key factors: surface antigens (agglutinogens) and antibodies (agglutinins).

Antigen   This is a protein the body recognises as being foreign. Surface antigens are on the erythrocytes.

Antibody   This is an immunoglobulin formed in response to an antigen. Antibodies are found in the plasma.

Agglutination   This is the clumping together and lysis of donated cells following a transfusion. It is termed an Antigen–Antibody Response. This will occur if incompatible blood is given. This will lead to the formation of emboli which will block capillaries, leading to ischaemia and death.

There are two major classifications of blood grouping (out of 300): **ABO and Rhesus.**

ABO System

Type	Surface antigens	Plasma antibodies
Type A	Agglutinogen A	Agglutinin b
Type B	Agglutinogen B	Agglutinin a
Type AB	Agglutinogens A & B	Neither agglutinin
Type O	Neither agglutinogen	Both agglutinins (a & b)

Rhesus factor   This is the presence of an antigen on red blood cells (RBC).

- Rhesus Positive (Rh+ve) — people who possess the antigen on RBC.
- Rhesus Negative (Rh-ve) — people who do not possess the antigen on RBC.

Normally, plasma does not contain an Antibody to Rhesus factor, but if exposed to Rhesus Antigen will manufacture Antibody and attack Rhesus Antigen at the next exposure.

BLOOD 2.3

Blood compatibility

Donor	Recipient			
	A Anti b	B Anti a	AB None	O Anti a & b
A	YES	NO	YES	NO
B	NO	YES	YES	NO
AB	NO	NO	YES	NO
O	YES	YES	YES	YES

Type O represents the **Universal donor**
Type AB represents the **Universal recipient**

Be aware of other agglutinogens and agglutinins in blood and the problems they can cause. Cross-matching should be done carefully.

Commonly used protocols for checking blood that is to be used for transfusion:

- Two nurses
- Patient's name, hospital number, date of birth
- Patient's blood group
- The correct blood product and number of units issued
- Blood unit number against blood transfusion request form
- Expiry date of blood unit
- Signatures of both nurses and entry in patient's records

Sources/bibliography: 1. O'Tool M, Keane CB. (1997) *Encyclopedia and Dictionary of Medicine, Nursing and Allied Health*, 6th edn. Philadelphia: WB Saunders. 2. Watson R. (2000) *Anatomy and Physiology for Nurses*, 11th edn. London: Harcourt. 3. Ross J, Wilson JW. (1990) *Anatomy and Physiology in Health and Illness*, 7th edn. London: Churchill Livingstone. 4. Hoffbrand AV, Pettit JE. (1994) *Essential Haematology*, 3rd edn. Oxford: Blackwell Science. 5. Bradbury M, Pope J. (1995) Blood and Blood Transfusion Reactions. *British Journal of Nursing*, Vol. 4, pp 814–17. 6. Glover G, Powell F. (1996) Blood Transfusion. *Nursing Standard*, Vol.10, pp 49–54. 7. Tortora GJ, Anagnostakos NP. (1987) *Principles of Anatomy and Physiology*, 5th edn. London: Harper & Row.

Risk of dangerous reactions associated with blood transfusion

Risk	Problem	Signs and symptoms
Fever	**Pyrogenic reaction:** waste products of bacterial activity in blood	Slight pyrexia
	White cells and platelet antibody: these also have antigens and can cause a reaction	Severe pyrexia
	Foreign protein antibody: rare to proteins in plasma	Severe pyrexia
	Infection: bacteria introduced into blood	Pyrexia, septicaemia, shock
Allergic reaction	Anti immunoglobulin A	If mild: pyrexia, skin rash, itching
	Antibodies react to immunoglobulin A protein in transfused blood	If severe: oedema and airway obstruction
Haemolytic reaction	This is caused by a major ABO incompatibility	Vein becomes heated, rapid pyrexia, chest feels constricted, dyspnoea, breathing rate increases, severe loin pain, shock (BP reduced, pulse increases, cold and clammy), headache, renal failure, disseminated intra-vascular coagulation (DIC)
Fluid overload	Generally only seen with groups who are already compromised cardiovascularly: older persons, young children	High blood pressure Pulmonary oedema Expectorating white frothy sputum Dyspnoea, confusion
Infection	Potential for introduction of bacteria and viruses such as: Pseudomonas, Staphylococcus	Pyrexia
Other risks associated with large blood transfusion	Hypothermia Cardiac arrythmias Adult respiratory distress syndrome (ARDS) Air embolism, hyperkalaemia	

Sources/bibliography: 1. Williamson LM, *et al.* (1998) *Serious Hazards of Transfusion.* Annual Report 1996–1997. Serious Hazards of Transfusion Scheme. Manchester: SHOT. 2. McClelland DBL. (ed.). Blood Transfusion Services of the United Kingdom. *Handbook of Transfusion Medicine*, 2nd edn. London: HMSO. 3. Place B. (1998) Blood Transfusion. *Nursing Times*, Vol 94, pp 48–50. 4. Mallett J, Dougherty L. (2000) *The Royal Marsden Hospital Manual of Clinical Nursing Procedures*, 5th edn. London: Blackwell Science. 5. Weinstein SH. (1997) *Plumer's Principles and Practice of Intravenous Therapy*, 6th edn. New York: JB Lippincott.

Physiological normal values

Measurement	Values		Notes
Pulse	130 bpm in newborn; 70–80 bpm adult; 60–80 bpm elderly		Check rhythm (regular or irregular)
Blood pressure	80/50	Normal newborn	All figures in mmHg **A good estimate of normal systolic BP is age in years + 100 as BP raises with age *WHO classification 1978 *Hypertension is only evident if figures are consistently raised
	120/70	Normal adult**	
	100 (systolic)	Hypotension	
	141/91 to 159/94*	Borderline hypertension*	
	160/95*	Hypertension*	
	30–40 mmHg	Pulse pressure	Difference between systolic and diastolic — low or high values give evidence of pathology
	5–12 cmH$_2$O	CVP	Manometer measurement in cmH$_2$O
	0 cm	JVP	Normally jugular veins are not filled at a 45° angle
Respiration	40–60	Normal newborn	Adult figures only Measured at rest
	10–20	Breaths per minute	
	420–500 ml	Tidal volume	
	7.5 l	Minute volume	
Temperature	Oral: 36°C to 37°C Axilla: 35.4°C to 36.4°C Tympanic: 36.8°C to 37.9°C Rectal: 36.6°C to 37.6°C In pyrexia, temperature will be 38°C or over (tympanic) In hypothermia, temperature will be 36°C or less (tympanic)		Rectal and tympanic temperature give most accurate reflection of core temperature Axilla is 0.6°C lower than oral whilst rectal is 0.6°C higher NB Children normally have a higher range (37.5–38°C) and the elderly may be lower (36.4°C tymp.) Diurnal and menstrual cycles affect body temperature

Sources/bibliography: 1. Marieb E. (2000) *Human Anatomy & Physiology*, 5th edn. California: Benjamin Cummings. 2. Cree L, Rischmiller S. (2000) *Science in Nursing*. Harcourt. Medline Encyclopedia at gov/medlineplus/ency/ encyclopedia_A-Ag.htm.

PHYSIOLOGICAL MONITORING 3.1

Measuring BP, CVP and JVP

Peripheral blood pressure (BP)

The sounds heard while measuring blood pressure using a sphygmomanometer are called the Korotkoff sounds, and have 5 phases:

1. initial 'tapping' sound (**cuff pressure = systolic pressure**)
2. sounds increase in intensity
3. sounds at maximum intensity
4. sounds become muffled
5. sounds disappear (**cuff pressure = diastolic pressure**)

Systolic pressure is registered as the pressure at which the sounds are first heard, and diastolic as the pressure at which they disappear (phase 5 of the Korotkoff sounds). NB. If you can palpate a radial pulse, the systolic blood pressure is usually at least 80 mmHg.

Central venous pressure (CVP)

Position the patient/manometer

-   Select an appropriate reference point for a CVP reading. This should be the sternal angle or mid-axilla point.
-   Mark the point on the patient and note in the medical/nursing record and CVP chart so that further measurements are taken from the identical point.

Set the scale to zero

-   Position the manometer so that the baseline is level with the right atrium (sternal angle or mid-axillary).
-   Loosen the scale fixing screw and slide the scale up or down until the baseline figure lies next to the arm of the spirit level representing a zero point.

Measuring the pressure

-   Flush the line with intravenous fluid (n/saline) allowing it to run through into the patient.
-   Turn off the three-way tap to the patient and allow it to fill from the IV bag; allow the manometer to fill slowly (do not let the fluid contact the filter at the top).
-   Turn off the three-way tap to the intravenous fluid bag and select the patient's CVP line as the fluid source.
-   The column of fluid should fall rapidly in the manometer.
-   The CVP reading is taken when the level of fluid in the manometer ceases to drop and oscillates with respiration.

Jugular venous pressure (JVP)

Position the patient

-   Position the patient at rest at a 45° recumbent angle (lay in bed and use backrest/pillows to prop the patient up).
-   Identify the top of the right clavicle as a landmark.
-   Identify the jugular vein on the right side of the patient's neck.

Measure the pressure

-   With the patient at 45°, estimate the jugular neck vein filling (distension and pulsation). Measure filling in cm vertically.
-   A jugular vein filled above the clavicle level at 45° is an indication of right heart volume overload. The level of filling (in cm) indicates the degree of overload.

Sources/bibliography: 1. Longmore JM, *et al.* (2000) *Oxford Handbook of Clinical Medicine.* Oxford: Oxford University Press. 2. Mallet J. (2000) *The Royal Marsden Hospital Manual of Clinical Nursing Procedures,* 5th edn. Blackwell. 3. Surgical Tutor at: http://www.surgical-tutor.org.uk/.

Fluid and electrolyte balance

Body water

Total body water = 42 l (approximately 60% of body weight)
25 l = intracellular (ICF): ~60%
17 l = extracellular (ECF): ~40%
- Plasma volume is 3–4 l (IVF): ~8%
- Extravascular volume is 11–13 l: (EVF) ~32%
  - Interstitial fluid (ISF): 10–12 l: ~30%
  - Transcellular water (TCW) is 400–600 ml: ~2% (joints, CSF, pleural cavity, peritoneal cavity, eye, GI secretions)

Balance

Daily fluid and electrolyte maintenance requirements vary for individuals. Intake must equal output. Loss increases with pyrexia, diarrhoea, vomiting, GI suction, ventilation, and polyurea with renal dysfunction. A good rule of thumb is for each 1°C of pyrexia an extra 1 l of fluid is required. NB This does not apply in renal dysfunction.

Intake: 24 hours

70 kg man: 2.5–3.0 l water, ~120–140 mmol sodium and 70 mmol potassium

40 kg woman: 2.0 l water, ~70–90 mmol sodium and 40 mmol potassium

Daily maintenance fluid requirements for children:
Weight 0–10 kg: 100 ml/kg
Weight 10–20 kg: 1000 ml + 50 ml/kg for each kg >10
Weight >20 kg: 1500 ml + 25 ml/kg for each kg >20

Output: 24 hours

Urine:	1400 ml (mandatory is 400–500 ml/24 hrs)
Sweat:	50 ml
Faecal:	150 ml
Insensible (lungs, skin):	800 ml

Sources/bibliography: 1. Hambly P. (2000) *Measuring the Blood Pressure*. http://www.nda.ox.ac.uk/wfsa/html/u11/u1106_01.htm#tpf. 2. The Centre for Disease Control and Prevention: http://www.cdc.gov/. 3. *Understanding Fluid Balance*: http://www.studentbmj.com/back issues/0497/data/0497ed1.htm. 4. *The Family Practitioners Notebook*. http://www.fpnotebook.com/.

PHYSIOLOGICAL MONITORING 3.3

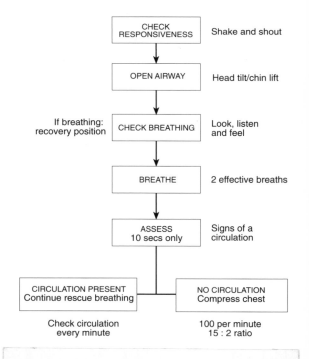

Basic life support algorithm

Adult basic life support

	CHECK RESPONSIVENESS	Shake and shout
	OPEN AIRWAY	Head tilt/chin lift
If breathing: recovery position	**CHECK BREATHING**	Look, listen and feel
	BREATHE	2 effective breaths
	ASSESS 10 secs only	Signs of a circulation

CIRCULATION PRESENT Continue rescue breathing	**NO CIRCULATION** Compress chest
Check circulation every minute	100 per minute 15 : 2 ratio

Send or go for help as soon as possible according to guidelines

For latest guidelines implemented from November 2005 refer to
http://www.resus.org.uk/SiteIndx.htm

RESUSCITATION 4.1

Anaphylaxis management in hospital

Anaphylactic reactions: treatment for adults by first medical responders

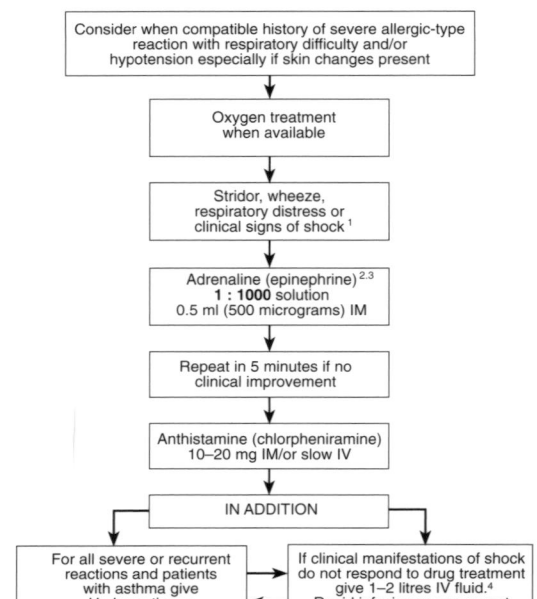

Consider when compatible history of severe allergic-type reaction with respiratory difficulty and/or hypotension especially if skin changes present

Oxygen treatment when available

Stridor, wheeze, respiratory distress or clinical signs of shock [1]

Adrenaline (epinephrine) [2,3]
1 : **1000** solution
0.5 ml (500 micrograms) IM

Repeat in 5 minutes if no clinical improvement

Anthistamine (chlorpheniramine) 10–20 mg IM/or slow IV

IN ADDITION

For all severe or recurrent reactions and patients with asthma give Hydrocortisone 100–500 mg IM/or slowly IV

If clinical manifestations of shock do not respond to drug treatment give 1–2 litres IV fluid. [4] Rapid infusion or one repeat dose may be necessary

1. An inhaled beta-agonist such as salbutamol may be used as an adjunctive measure if bronchospasm is severe and does not respond rapidly to other treatment.

2. If profound shock judged *immediately* life-threatening, give CPR/ALS if necessary. Consider *slow* IV adrenaline (epinephrine) 1 : 10 000 solution. This is hazardous and is recommended only for an experienced practitioner who can also obtain IV access without delay. Note the different strength of adrenaline (epinephrine) that may be required for IV use.

3. If adults are treated with an Epipen, the 300 micrograms will usually be sufficient. A second dose may be required. Half doses of adrenaline (epinephrine) may be safer for patients on amitriptyline, imipramine, or beta blocker.

4. A crystalloid may be safer than a colloid.

RESUSCITATION 4.2

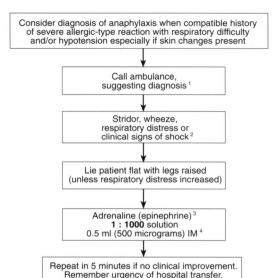

Anaphylaxis management in the community

Anaphylactic reactions: treatment for adults in the community

Consider diagnosis of anaphylaxis when compatible history of severe allergic-type reaction with respiratory difficulty and/or hypotension especially if skin changes present

↓

Call ambulance, suggesting diagnosis [1]

↓

Stridor, wheeze, respiratory distress or clinical signs of shock [2]

↓

Lie patient flat with legs raised (unless respiratory distress increased)

↓

Adrenaline (epinephrine) [3]
1 : 1000 solution
0.5 ml (500 micrograms) IM [4]

↓

Repeat in 5 minutes if no clinical improvement. Remember urgency of hospital transfer.

1. Ambulance will be equipped with oxygen, salbutamol and fluids which may be used as adjunctive therapy.

2. If profound shock judged to be *immediately* life-threatening, give CPR/ALS if necessary.

3. Half doses of adrenaline (epinephrine) may be safer for patients on amitriptyline, imipramine, or beta blocker.

4. If adults are treated with an Epipen, the 300 micrograms will usually be sufficient. A second dose may be required, but this should be considered ONLY if the patient's condition continues to deteriorate 5 minutes after the first dose

   NB *Remember the urgency of hospital transfer.*

RESUSCITATION 4.3

Management of choking

Management of choking in adults

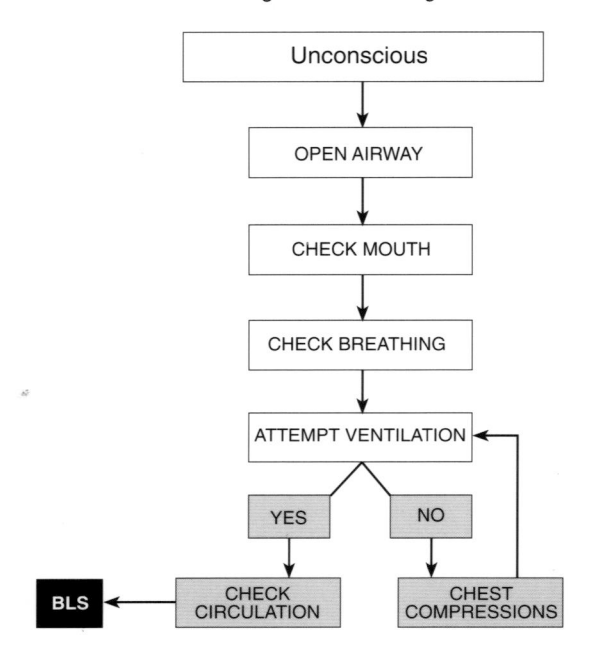

Sources/bibliography: 1. Project Team of the Resuscitation Council (UK) (1999). Emergency medical treatment of anaphylactic reactions. *J Accid Emerg Med*, Vol 16: pp 243–8.

RESUSCITATION 4.4

Reading ECGs

Electrocardiography: graphic representation of the electrical currents generated within the heart, detected at the skin surface

The cycle of electrical currents have been identified by the letters PQRST

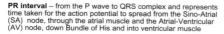

**UK standard ECG rate =
25mm/second: 'big square' = 0.2 seconds
'small square' = 0.04 seconds**

To calculate the rate: count the number of big squares between two consecutive QRS complexes and divide this into 300

P – represents atrial activation
QRS – represents ventricular activation
T – represents recovery of ventricular muscle

PR interval – from the P wave to QRS complex and represents time taken for the action potential to spread from the Sino-Atrial (SA) node, through the atrial muscle and the Atrial-Ventricular (AV) node, down Bundle of His and into ventricular muscle

QRS complex – time taken for action potential to pass through the ventricles

ST segment – flat line between S and T waves, represents early recovery of ventricular muscle

Reading a Rhythm Strip: the golden rules

1. Is there any electrical activity?
Check: all leads, size button and electrical connections.
A completely straight line suggests a technical fault. Asystole is never a straight line as it is distorted by baseline drift, respiratory movement or resuscitation

2. What is the ventricular (QRS) rate?
Normal heart rate is 60–100 bpm
Bradycardia = <60, Tachycardia = >100
To determine the rate divide 300 by the number of big squares between QRS complexes

3. Is the QRS rhythm regular?
Compare R–R intervals at different places in the recording

4. Is the QRS complex width normal or prolonged?
Normal maximum width for QRS is 3 small squares

5. Is atrial activity present?
Is there a P wave?

6. How is atrial activity related to ventricular activity?
Is the time interval between P wave and QRS consistent?
Is there a P wave for every QRS?

ECG INTERPRETATION 5.1

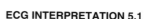

Useful cardiac arrhythmias

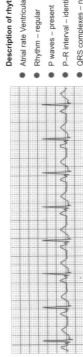

Description of rhythm: sinus rhythm

- Atrial rate Ventricular rate 100
- Rhythm – regular
- P waves – present
- P–R interval – identifiable
- QRS complexes – normal

Description of rhythm: atrial fibrillation

- Atrial rate >360 min
- Ventricular rate 60–160 min
- Rhythm – totally regular
- P waves – none seen
- P–R interval – not identifiable
- QRS complexes – normal

Clinical features

May be caused by :

- increased sympathetic tone
- atrial muscle damage
- congestive cardiac failure
- normally not associated with drop in blood pressure

Useful cardiac arrhythmias

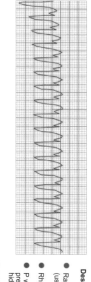

Description of rhythm: ventricular tachycardia

- Rate – 150 bpm
  (usually 140–220 bpm)

- Rhythm – slightly regular

- P waves – usually
  present but may be
  hidden in QRS complex

- PR interval – not
  identifiable

- QRS complexes – wide

Clinical features

May be caused by :

- Ischaemic heart disease

- Hypoxia, acidosis, low
  potassium

- If rate is above 120–140 blood
  pressure is likely to be low
  leading to poor tissue perfusion

- May lead to VF and death

Description of rhythm: ventricular fibrillation

- Rate – unclear

- Rhythm – irregular

- P waves – unrecognisable

- PR interval – absent

- QRS complexes absent

Clinical features

Causes: see above

- Will lead to cardiac arrest

ECG INTERPRETATION 5.3

Useful cardiac arrhythmias

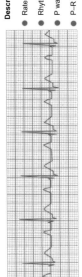

Description of rhythm: 1st degree heart block

- Rate – normal
- Rhythm – regular
- P waves – normal
- P–R interval wide
- QRS complex – normal

Clinical features

- May be caused by damage to AV node, hypoxia, drugs overdose
- No effect on patient if the rate is normal

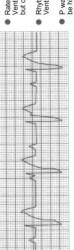

Description of rhythm: 3rd degree heart block

- Rate – atria normal
  Ventricular rate is 60 bpm but can be 20–50 bpm
- Rhythm – atria are regular
  Ventricles usually regular
- P waves – normal but can be hidden
- PR interval absent
- QRS complex – abnormal width may vary

Clinical features

- May be caused by damage to AV node, bundle of His or bundle branches (ischaemic disease)
- If ventricular rate low, blood pressure may be reduced

Sources/bibliography: 1. Shuldham C. (1998) *Cardiorespiratory Nursing*.
Cheltenham: Stanley Thornes Publishers Ltd. 2. Alexander MF, Fawcett JN,
Runciman PJ. (1999) *Nursing Practice – Hospital and Home – The Adult*.
London: Churchill Livingstone. 3. Paz J, Panik M. (1997) *Acute Care Handbook
for Physical Therapists*. Oxford: Butterworth-Heinemann. 4. Corke C. (2000)
Practical Intensive Care Medicine – Problem Solving in the ICU. Oxford:
Butterworth-Heinemann. 5. Moulton C, Yates D. (1999) *Emergency Medicine*.
Oxford: Blackwell Science. 6. Goldhill D, Withington P. (1997) *Textbook of
Intensive Care*. London: Chapman and Hall Medical. 7. Ryan D, Park C. (1995)
Colour Atlas of Critical and Intensive Care – Diagnosis and Investigation.
London: Mosby-Wolfe.

Daily nutritional requirements

Average daily nutritional requirements for an adult

Nutrient	Amount required
Energy (mostly from carbohydrate, only 20% should be from fat)	8.4 MJ
Protein	~50 g (0.8 g/kg body weight)
Fluid and electrolytes	
Water	2600 ml
Sodium	80 mmol
Potassium	70 mmol
Chloride	105 mmol
Phosphate	13 mmol
Calcium	10 mmol
Magnesium	10 mmol
Trace elements	
Iron	0.18 mmol
Copper	0.04 mmol
Zinc	0.30 mmol
Manganese	0.02 mmol
Vitamins (water soluble)	
Thiamine (B_1)	1.4 mg
Riboflavin (B_2)	2.1 mg
Pyridoxine (B_6)	2.1 mg
Cyanocobalamine (B_{12})	2.0 mg
Nicotinamide	14 mg
Biotin	0.4 mg
Folic acid	2 mg
Ascorbic acid (C)	35 mg

These figures will vary with individuals and metabolism. For example older people will need less protein and more vitamins, whilst children, athletes and patients with wounds will require more protein.

CLINICAL ASSESSMENT AND MANAGEMENT 6.1

Daily nutritional requirements

Vitamins (fat soluble)	
Calciferol (D)	100 IU
Phytylmenaquinone (K)	140 mg
Retinol (A)	700 IU
Tocopheryl acetate (E)	30 IU

Typical enteral feeds and nutritional supplements	
Clinifeed	Protein, carbohydrate, fat, vitamins and minerals; gluten free
Ensure	Protein, carbohydrate, fat, vitamins and minerals, trace elements; gluten and lactose free
Entera	Protein, carbohydrate, fat, vitamins and minerals, trace elements; gluten and lactose free
Fresubin	Protein, carbohydrate, fat, vitamins and minerals, trace elements; gluten and lactose free
Provide	Protein, carbohydrate; gluten and lactose free
Elemental 028	Protein, carbohydrate, fat, vitamins and minerals, trace elements

Body Mass Index (BMI)

BMI is a scientific measure that uses your height and weight. You can calculate BMI by dividing weight in kilograms by the square of your height in meters.

The algebraic expression for BMI is: $BMI = kg/(m)^2$

BMI <20 indicates a lean BMI/low amount of body fat
BMI 20–22 indicates the ideal, healthy amount of body fat
BMI 23–25 is still within an acceptable range
BMI 26–30 indicates an excess of body fat
BMI >30 indicates obesity

N.B. BMI fails to consider lean body mass. It is possible for a healthy, muscular individual with very low body fat to be classified obese using the BMI formula.

Sources/bibliography: 1. Shami S, Davidson T. (1997) Understanding fluid balance. 2. Whitney EN. (ed.) (1997) Understanding Normal and Clinical Nutrition, Wadsworth. 1 & 2. *Student BMJ*, Vol. 5, London. 3. Surgical Tutor at: http://www.surgical-tutor.org.uk.

CLINICAL ASSESSMENT AND MANAGEMENT 6.2

Pressure area care

Definition: lesions caused by unrelieved pressure against soft tissue, usually over bony prominences (*National Pressure Ulcer Advisory Panel*). Pressure sores result from an interruption of the tissue's blood supply causing local ischaemia; if this is allowed to continue tissue necrosis will follow.

Factors contributing to pressure area breakdown: compression of tissues, shearing force, heat, moisture, friction, poor skin hygiene, poor general nutrition, lack of oxygen, lack of spontaneous body movements, age, medical condition.

Grading of pressure sores
1. Non-blanchable erythema, redness that remains present over an area under pressure 30 minutes after pressure source is removed. Skin intact.
2. Epidermis is broken, superficial lesion, no measurable depth. Partial thickness skin loss.
3. Full thickness skin loss down through dermis, may include subcutaneous tissue, may undermine adjacent tissue.
4. Full thickness skin loss extending into supportive structures, e.g. muscle, tendon and bone. May undermine and have various sinus tracts.

Treatment and prevention
The most effective treatments for and prevention of pressure area breakdown include:
- Frequent turning or moving the patient (e.g. at least 2 hourly)
- Avoiding leaving patients on inappropriate surfaces (e.g. trolley) for any longer than essential
- Keeping bed linen crease-free
- Using an air or foam mattress
- Keeping the skin clean and dry
- Ensuring adequate nutrition/hydration
- A multidisciplinary approach is the most effective (OT/PT/dietician).

1. Occiput
2. Spinous processes
3. Scapula
4. Shoulder
5. Elbow
6. Sacrum
7. Iliac crest
8. Ischial tuberosity
9. Knee
10. Heel
11. Side of foot

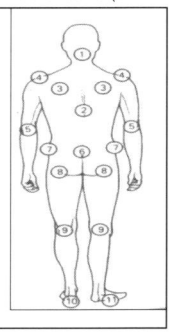

Risk assessment: assessment tools consider both extrinsic and intrinsic factors that contribute to a change in skin integrity. There are a number of scales that have been developed to identify those at risk of developing pressure sores. The Waterlow scale has been identified as more accurate in predicting formation of pressure sores. However, while assessment of risk is essential, the reliability and validity of an assessment tool should not be taken for granted.

CLINICAL ASSESSMENT AND MANAGEMENT 6.3

Decubitus ulcer assessment

The Waterlow Scale (Adapted from Waterlow 1991)

Build/weight for height		Skin type/visual risk areas		Sex/age	
Average	1	Healthy	0	Male	1
Above average	2	Tissue paper	2	Female	2
Obese	3	Dry	1	14–49	1
Below	4	Oedematous	1	50–64	2
		Clammy	1	65–74	3
		Discoloured	2	75–80	4
		Broken	3	81+	5

Continence		Mobility		Neurological deficit	
Complete/cath	0	Fully	0	Diabetes/MS/CVA	
Occasionally incont	1	Restless	1	motor/sensory	
Cath/incont faeces	2	Apathetic	2	paraplegia	4–6
Doubly incontinent	3	Restricted	3		
		Inert/traction	4		
		Chairbound	5		

Major surgery/trauma		Medication		Special risks	
Orthopaedic:		Cytotoxics		Tissue malnutrition	
below waist/spinal	5	high dose	4	terminal cachexia	8
on table >2 hours	5	Steroids		Cardiac failure	5
		anti-inflammatory		Peripheral vascular	
				disease	5
				Anaemia	2
				Smoking	1

Score:
10+ at risk
13+ high risk   *several scores can be used per category*
20+ very high risk

Sources/bibliography: 1. Waterlow J. (1998) The Treatment and Use of the Waterlow Card. *Nursing Times*, Vol. 94: pp 63–7. 2. Mallett J, Dougherty L. (eds) (2000) *Manual of Clinical Nursing Procedures*. Royal Marsden Hospital. Oxford: Blackwell Science. 3. Phipps W, Cassmeyer V, Sands J, Lehman M. (1995) *Medical Surgical Nursing. Concepts and Clinical Practice*, 5th edn. St Louis, Missouri: Mosby. 4. Roper N, Logan W, Tierney A. (1999) *The Elements of Nursing*. A Model for Nursing Based on a Model of Living, 4th edn. London: Churchill Livingstone.

Phlebitis assessment

Definition of phlebitis

Phlebitis is the acute inflammation of the intima of the vein.

Causes

- Mechanical abrasion
- Hypertonic solutions or acid/alkali drugs/solutions
- Particulate matter in IV solution (mainly due to in-line drug additions)
- Bacterial contamination (rare)

Prevention

- Stringent aseptic technique and use of in-line IV filters
- Re-siting of cannulae after 48 hours
- Avoid peripheral administration of irritant solutions (e.g. TPN, acid or alkali drugs)

Treatment

- Re-site cannulae immediately
- If infection suspected, use of prescribed antibiotic therapy
- The use of Ichthammol bandage, although mildly antiseptic, has unproven efficacy

Phlebitis grading

0 = no clinical symptoms
1+ = erythema with or without pain; oedema may or may not be present; no palpable venous cord
2+ = erythema with or without pain; oedema may or may not be present; streak formation; no palpable cord
3+ = erythema with or without pain; oedema may or may not be present; streak formation; palpable cord

Infiltration grading

1 = skin blanched, oedema <1", cool to touch, with or without pain
2 = skin blanched, oedema 1–6", cool to touch, with or without pain
3 = skin blanched (may be translucent), oedema >6", cool to touch, mild to moderate pain and possible numbness
4 = skin blanched, translucent, tight and leaking, oedema >6", deep pitting tissue oedema, circulatory impairment

Sources/bibliography: 1. The Intravenous Nurses Society. (1998) Revised intravenous nursing standards of practice. *J Intravenous Nursing*, Vol 21, pp 48, 50–9, 63. 2. The Intravenous Nurses Society. (1998) *Handbook of Infusion Therapy*. Springhouse, PA: Springhouse Corp. 3. The Intravenous Nurses Society, Fresh Pond Sq, 10 Fawcett Street, Cambridge, MA 02138; or visit www.ins1.org.

Stool assessment

The Bristol Stool Form Scale

Type 1		Separate hard lumps, like nuts (hard to pass) (CONSTIPATED STOOL)
Type 2		Sausage-shaped but lumpy
Type 3		Like a sausage but with cracks on its surface
Type 4		Like a sausage or snake, smooth and soft
Type 5		Soft blobs with clear-cut edges (passed easily)
Type 6		Fluffy pieces with ragged edges, a mushy stool
Type 7		Watery, no solid pieces ENTIRELY LIQUID (DIARRHOEA)

The Bristol Stool Chart is commonly used to describe the type and consistency of stool. Reproduced with kind permission from Dr KW Heaton.

Constipation/laxatives

Definition: The passage of hard stools less frequently than the patient's own normal pattern.

The first stage when considering the use of laxatives is to establish if the patient is constipated and that the constipation is not a result of an undiagnosed, underlying complaint. A thorough assessment is required and it is essential to determine what is 'normal' for the patient when discussing bowel movements.

Increasing the amount of dietary fibre normally relieves simple constipation. Prolonged treatment of constipation is rarely required, except occasionally in the elderly.

CLINICAL ASSESSMENT AND MANAGEMENT 6.6

Laxatives

Laxatives can be divided into four main groups:

1. Bulk forming laxatives

Increase faecal mass that in turn stimulates peristalsis.

Indications: constipation. **Route**: oral. **Patient education**: patients should be informed that it may take a few days for the full effect to develop.

Cautions: ensure adequate fluid intake to avoid intestinal obstruction.

Examples: ispaghula husk granules, methylcellulose and sterculia preparations.

Note: long-term use in those with uncomplicated constipation.

2. Stimulant laxatives

Increase intestinal motility.

Indications: constipation. **Route**: oral. **Patient education**: patients should be informed that they may experience abdominal cramp.

Cautions: not to be used in intestinal obstruction. Prolonged use may precipitate the onset of atonic non-functioning colon and hypokalaemia. Co-danthramer and co-danthrusate are only licensed for prophylaxis and relief of constipation in terminally ill patients of all ages (potential human carcinogen).

Examples: bisocodyl, senna, co-danthramer and co-danthrusate.

Note: functional constipation that is resistant to dietary measures.

3. Faecal softeners

Lubricate and soften impacted faeces and promote a bowel action.

Indications: constipation. **Route**: rectal (enema/suppositories) containing arachis oil (ground nut oil, peanut oil).

Patient education: explain the procedure to the patient. Maintain patient dignity at all times. Observe and follow usual procedure for administration of enemas (see local guidelines). May cause local irritation.

Examples: glycerine suppositories, arachis oil enema.

4. Osmotic laxatives

Retain fluid in the bowel by osmosis or by changing the pattern of water distribution in the faeces, thus increasing stool weight and stimulating colonic movement.

Indications: constipation. **Route**: oral/rectal (enema).

Patient education: osmotic laxatives may cause cramps, flatulence and abdominal discomfort. Enemas may cause local irritation. Explain the procedure to the patient. Maintain patient dignity at all times. Observe and follow usual procedure for administration of enemas (see local guidelines).

Examples: (a) oral lactulose, (b) rectal (enema) phosphates.

Note: generally reserved for second line laxatives when others have failed.

Caution: avoided in patients with colitis/ inflamed haemorrhoids or skin tags/ acute gastrointestinal conditions/anal or rectal surgical wounds or trauma/ those who have recently had radiotherapy to the lower pelvic area/the elderly and debilitated/proctitis/inflammatory bowel conditions.

Sources/bibliography: 1. *Nurses Prescribing Formulary 1999-2001*. Royal Pharmaceutical Society of Great Britain. 2. Addison R. (2000) How to Administer Enemas and Suppositories. Continence NT Plus. *Nursing Times*, Vol 96: pp 3–4. 3. Butler M. (1998) Laxatives and Rectal Preparations. *Nursing Times*, Vol 94, pp 56–8.

Catheter types and sizes

Catheter materials

Catheters are available in a range of materials. The material used determines how long the catheter can stay in the bladder:

- **Short term** (7–14 days) plastic (PVC), latex
- **Medium term** (up to 28 days) Teflon coated latex
- **Long term** (up to 12 weeks) all silicone, silicone elastomer coated latex, hydrogel coated latex

Sizes

Using the correct size of catheter is crucial to the success of the procedure. The system of measurement used to express external catheter diameter is the Charrière (Ch).

1 Ch = 1/3 mm diameter 12 Ch = 4 mm diameter

The correct size is the smallest possible size for providing adequate drainage. If too large a diameter is selected it can cause urethral irritation and subsequent damage. The following guide can be used:

Female 12/13 Ch   **Male** 12/14/16 Ch

If the patient is having problems with their catheter drainage, do not assume a larger size is required. This may have an adverse effect, causing irritation and leading to bypassing. Catheters over 18 Ch are rarely required and their use should always be questioned.

Balloon sizes

There are three different sizes of balloon:

1. 5 ml paediatric balloon
2. 10 ml for routine drainage
3. 30 ml or larger specifically for postoperative use

Excess water may lead to dragging of the catheter; it can also cause bladder spasm and discomfort.
Sterile water should be used to fill the balloon.

Length

Catheters come in three lengths:

1. Paediatric (for children)
2. Female 26 cm female catheters are shorter than male catheters due to shorter urethra
3. Male (standard) 43 cm

Tips and eyes

There are many tips available; in most cases a straight tip should be selected. Catheters usually have two eyes.

Sources/bibliography: 1. National Prescribing Centre (1999). *Prescribing Factsheet 20.* 2. *You and Your Catheter.* Tubiton House, Oldham: Seton Continence Care (set 3106). 3. *Management and Care of Catheters and Collection Systems*: A Guide for Nurses. Forest House, Crawley: Bard Ltd.

CLINICAL ASSESSMENT AND MANAGEMENT 6.8

Infection classification

Exogenous infection: patients become infected with organisms from the external environment.

Endogenous infection: from patients' own internal organisms (especially immunocompromised patients).

Nosocomial infection: hospital acquired infection (HAI). Defined as an infection that is neither present nor incubating before hospital admission. In hospital, potential sources of infection include: patients, personnel, visitors, equipment, linen, etc. The most common route of infection is by direct contact, most frequently on the hands of staff. Handwashing is acknowledged to be the main activity for preventing the spread of nosocomial infection.

Prevention of infection

Exogenous

Medical/nursing staff:

- Do not provide care when ill
- Check immunisations are current
- Effective handwashing
- Use gloves when handling any body substances.

Other areas:

- Do not shake or put bed linen on floor
- Proper disposal of waste
- Cleansing and sterilisation of contaminated articles
- Ventilation: negative pressure in single rooms to prevent air leaving room
- Effective mopping and damp dusting.

Endogenous

- Patient education regarding good nutrition/personal hygiene (especially handwashing)
- Antibiotics and chemotherapy affect the normal flora of the patient allowing colonisation. Ensure antibiotics are given as and when directed. Patient education: need for completing course and only taking when prescribed by physician.

Recipients of care—psychological effects of isolation. Research has shown that isolated patients are significantly more anxious and depressed than other hospitalised patients. The reasons for this include fear of the unknown and loss of control. This is compounded by reduced contact and communication with health-care professionals and friends/family due to isolation procedures. Measures to meet the psychological needs of the isolated patient should be a key part of the assessment process.

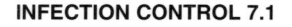

Universal precautions

Definition: routine safe working practices adopted to protect staff and patients from infection by blood and body fluids.

Health care workers frequently come into contact with blood, secretions and excreta. This means that they may be exposed to pathogens including blood-borne viruses such as HIV and hepatitis B+C. As it is impossible to identify all those with infection, it is recommended that all body fluids be treated as potentially infectious and universal precautions followed.

Handwashing: must be carried out after removal of protective clothing, between each patient contact, after contact with blood or any body fluids, before any invasive procedures and before handling food.

Skin: abrasions should be covered with a waterproof dressing which is breathable and an effective viral and bacterial barrier.

Gloves: seamless, non-powdered gloves should be worn when contact with body fluids is anticipated.

Aprons: disposable plastic aprons should be worn when splashing with body fluids is anticipated.

Eye protection: goggles or safety spectacles should be worn when splashing with body fluids or other debris is anticipated.

Masks: water-repellent masks should be worn if there is a risk of blood or body fluids splashing the face.

Sharps: dispose of used sharps at the point of use into an approved sharps container. Do not resheath needles or over-fill sharps containers.

Needlestick injury: 1. Encourage bleeding from wound site. 2. Wash thoroughly with soap and water. 3. Cover with waterproof dressing. 4. Note the name of patient if known. 5. Report to Occupational Health. 6. Complete incident form and report to line manager. 7. If patient is thought to be HIV positive, seek Occupational Health for advice/consideration of Post Exposure Prophylaxis (follow PEP guidelines).

Conjunctivae/mucous membranes: if splashed by blood or body fluids, irrigate with copious amount of saline (follow steps from 4 above).

Waste: all waste with blood or body fluids must be placed in yellow clinical waste sacks and sent for incineration (refer to local policy).

Sources/bibliography: 1. Mallett J, Dougherty L. (eds) (2000) *Manual of Clinical Nursing Procedures*. Royal Marsden Hospital. Oxford: Blackwell Science. 2. Roper N, Logan W, Tierney A. (1999) *The Elements of Nursing*. A Model for Nursing Based on a Model of Living, 4th edn. London: Churchill Livingstone. 3. Phipps W, Cassmeyer V, Sands J, Lehman M. (1995) *Medical Surgical Nursing. Concepts and Clinical Practice*, 5th edn. St Louis, Missouri: Mosby. 4. Oakley K. (1994) Making Sense of Universal Precautions. *Nursing Times*, Vol 90: pp 35–6. 5. Royal College of Nursing. (2000) *Working Well Initiative*, Universal Precautions for the Control of Infection. RCN. 6. Royal College of Nursing. (2001) *Working Well Initiative*, Good Practice in Infection Control. RCN.

Barrier nursing

Definition: the use of infection control practices aimed at controlling the spread of, and destroying, pathogenic organisms. This may require mechanical barriers to contain organisms within a specified area.

Barrier nursing includes:

1. Source isolation to segregate infected patients in single rooms to prevent the spread of infection.

2. Group source isolation to segregate a number of patients with the same infection in one ward (if there are not enough single rooms to prevent spread of infection).

3. Strict source isolation to segregate patients infected with a serious contagious disease in isolation units to prevent the spread of infection, e.g. viral haemorrhagic fever. Requirements for source isolation include: (a) an anteroom for protective clothing; (b) handwashing facilities; (c) toilet facilities. The most important measures are handwashing and protection of clothes (gowns, caps, masks).

4. Protective isolation (reverse barrier nursing) to keep immunosuppressed patients separate to protect them from acquiring an exogenous infection.

Spread of infection in hospitals (Adapted from Roper, Logan, Tierney (1999)).

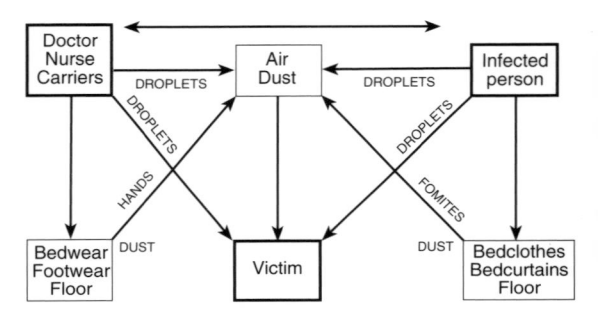

Care providers: health-care staff who perform clinical procedures should be aware of, and adhere to, written procedure guidance from their employer. Risk assessment is essential for each procedure to prevent, control or limit the risk to staff.

SI units

Amount	=	moles
		amount of substance
Length	=	metres, m
		centimetres, cm
Area	=	metres^2, m^2
Volume	=	litres, l
		millilitres, ml
Weight	=	newtons, N
Mass	=	kilograms, kg
		grams, g
		milligrams, mg
		micrograms, mcg or µg
Atomic mass	=	daltons or AMU

Notes:

The actual weight of an object is represented by its mass × gravity and is measured in newtons. The term 'weight' however is commonly used to describe mass and is acceptable for objects within the Earth's atmosphere.

The mass of 1 cm^3 of pure water (1 ml) is 1 g. Therefore, 1 litre of pure water weighs 1 kg.

Prefixes for SI units

Prefix	Abbreviation	Factor	
tera-	T	10^{12}	= million million
giga-	G	10^9	= thousand million
mega-	M	10^6	= million
kilo-	k	10^3	= thousand
hecto-	h	10^2	= hundred
deca- or deka-	da	10	= ten
deci-	d	10^{-1}	= tenth
centi-	c	10^{-2}	= hundredth
milli-	m	10^{-3}	= thousandth
micro-	mc or µ	10^{-6}	= millionth
nano-	n	10^{-9}	= thousand millionth

The logarithmic scale for acidity/alkalinity

A logarithm is the exponent or power to which a stated number, called the base, is raised to yield a specific number. For example, in the expression $10^2 = 100$ the logarithm of 100 is 2 (for the base 10), i.e. 10 x 10 =100. Each step of this logarithmic scale multiplies the preceding step by 10 (the exception being 0), e.g.

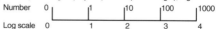

Positive logs describe very large numbers and negative logs very small numbers. A negative log is given the expression p. Negative logs are used in the calculation of acidity/alkalinity as this is a measure of the concentration of hydrogen ions (H$^+$) in solution (a very small amount). This is therefore known as pH. An **acidic solution with a pH of 6** contains 10^{-6} mole/l of hydrogen ions (0.000001 mole/l) whereas an **alkaline solution with a pH of 8** contains 10^{-8} mole/l of hydrogen ions (0.00000001 mole/l) i.e. it has a hundred times less H$^+$ ions in it than the pH 6 solution.

DRUG ADMINISTRATION 8.1

Calculating dosage/delivery

Here are two simple ways that you can use to check the correct drug dose:

A. Use the formula:

$$\frac{\text{Dose prescribed}}{\text{Units in which the drug is available}} \times \text{Dose available}$$

e.g. 20 mg of frusemide is prescribed and the ward stock is 5 mg tablets

$$\frac{20 \text{ mg}}{5 \text{ mg}} \times 1 \text{ tablet} = 4 \text{ tablets}$$

B. Find the dosage in the smallest unit available and divide the prescribed dose by this figure.

e.g. 10 mg of temazepam is prescribed and the ward stock is 25 mg in 20 ml elixir

The smallest single unit is 1 ml

Divide 25 mg by 20 ml to find out the dosage per ml = 1.25 mg per ml

Therefore the dosage is

$$\frac{10}{1.25} = 8 \text{ ml}$$

IV fluid infusion rates for fluids with gravity feed drip sets

When you need to calculate an IV infusion rate, you need to know the following information:

1. prescription giving volume of fluid to be infused and time over which it is to be given, e.g. 1 litre of saline over 8 hours.

2. if you are using a gravity drip-giving set, you will need to know the number of drops in the giving set which make up 1 ml. This is written on the packaging. (N.B. normally 20 macrodrops = 1 ml crystalloid and 15 macrodrops = 1 ml colloid; e.g. 20 drops of H_2O = 1 ml).

Then calculate the following:

1. The number of ml to be given per minute
2. Multiply this figure by the number of drops in 1 ml

e.g. for 1 litre of saline over 8 hours

1000 ml/8 hours = 125 ml/hour
125 ml/60 mins = 2.08 ml/min
2.08 ml/min × 20 drops/ml = 41.6 drops per minute

This is closest to 42 drops per minute so you would run the infusion at a 42-drops-per-minute rate.

N.B. If you need to be very accurate in your IV fluid administration, USE A PUMP OR CONTROLLER not a gravity feed system!

Drug delivery in infusions

Where drugs are to be given by IV infusion, **a pump or controller should always be used**, unless it is a small volume to be infused over a short period, e.g. metronidazole 500 mg in 100 ml given over 30 minutes.

When you need to calculate an IV drug infusion rate, you need to know the following:

1. The concentration of the drug solution in your stock
2. The volume of the drug to be infused
3. The time over which the drug is to be infused

Then work out the following:

1. The prescribed amount of the drug to be infused per hour
2. The dose of the drug per ml of the infusion
3. The number of ml of the infusion to be given per hour

Here is an example:

An isorbide dinitrate infusion at 4 mg per hour is prescribed.
The ward stock of this drug is 5 mg in 10 ml.

Therefore, the dose of the drug per ml of the infusion is:
$$\frac{5 \text{ mg}}{10 \text{ ml}} = 0.5 \text{ mg/ml}$$

So if you divide the prescribed dose per hour by the dose per ml you get the required ml per hour:
$$\frac{4 \text{ mg/hour}}{0.5 \text{ mg/ml}} = 8 \text{ ml per hour}$$

It may often be necessary to dilute a drug in a fluid (usually normal saline) in order to give the infusion.

Here is an example:

An actrapid insulin infusion is prescribed at 5 units per hour.
The ward stock of actrapid insulin is 100 units in 1 ml and the only pump device available is a 50 ml syringe pump.

Therefore, a 50 ml syringe is filled with N/saline and then 0.5 ml is expelled. Then 0.5 ml (50 units) of actrapid insulin is added.

This gives us a solution of 1 unit of insulin per ml, and can be set to run at 5 ml/hour.

$$\frac{5 \text{ units/hour}}{1 \text{ unit/ml}} = 5 \text{ ml/hour}$$

Calculating IV doses using weight

Occasionally, you may come across a prescription for infusion using a patient's weight. This is best illustrated by an example:

> Dobutamine at 4 mcg/kg/minute is prescribed.
>
> This means giving a dobutamine infusion at a rate of 4 mcg per kg of the patient's weight per minute.

First, you need to know the patient's weight.

> The patient weighs 65 kg

Then simply multiply the dose by the patient's weight to find out the correct dose per minute for this patient's weight.

> $4 \times 65 = 260$ mcg/minute

Then multiply the dose per minute by 60 (minutes) to give you the total dose per hour.

> $260 \times 60 = 15600$ mcg/hour = 15.6 mg/hour

Golden rules for drug calculation

1. Always ensure that you are working with the same units in your calculations. Convert units if necessary to achieve this.

   i.e. **mg or mcg but not both together!**

2. Always look at your result from a drug calculation and ask: is this a reasonable dose?

   i.e. a 600 g dose of antibiotics or a 20 tablet dose of frusemide are both likely to be incorrect!

3. If working out a complex dose calculation or if you are ever unsure, always get someone to check your result.

Sources/bibliography: 1. Ogden SJ, Radcliff RK. (1999) *The Calculation of Drug Dosages.* Mosby. 2. Bayt PT. (1999) *Administering Medications,* 4th edn. New York: Glencoe/McGraw-Hill. 3. Utton BM. (1998) Nursing mathematics: the importance of application. *Nursing Standard,* Vol 13: pp 35–8. 4. The University of Kansas. *Clinical Experience Drug Dosage* web site at: http://www2.kumc.edu/instruction/ nursing/n420/clinical/CalculatingDrugDosages.html. 5. *A Model for Safe Medication Administration in Hospitals* at: http://www.fha.org/acrobat/ administrationrevised2901.pdf. 6. UKCC *Guidelines for the Administration of Medicines* at: http://www.ukcc.org.uk/cms/content/Publications/ Guidelines%20for%20medicines%20.pdf.

IV Therapy: cannula selection

Choice of device

Selection of the appropriate cannula is important for the success of IV therapy and patient comfort.

Variations in cannulae design

Three distinct product materials exist: steel needles, PTFE catheters and polyurethane catheters. Steel needles are only suitable for very short-term use during the administration of non-irritant products. Polyurethane catheters may be designed with thinner walls, thereby producing a greater flow rate compared to an equivalent PTFE catheter and it is suggested that polyurethane materials may reduce the incidence of infusion phlebitis.

Design variations include:

Design variations include:

- thickness of cannula needle wall
- sharpness and angle of heel
- properties: steel and Teflon do not soften; Neoflon expands, becoming larger in the vein giving greater flow; and Vialon softens, becoming more pliable
- safety features to prevent blood contact

The cannula chosen should be as small as possible for the task. This allows a good blood circulation around the device, reducing the risk of thrombophlebitis.

Colour/size Int. diameter/length Flow ml/min Use		
Brown		
14		
1.6 mm/45 mm		
315		
Blood/ trauma/ high volumes		
Grey		
16		
1.4 mm/45 mm		
180		
As above		
Green		
18		
1.0 mm/45 mm		
80		
Fluids & blood products		

Colour/size Int. diameter/length Flow ml/min Use		
Pink		
20		
0.8 mm/32 mm		
54		
Up to 3 litres a day of fluids		
Blue		
22		
0.6 mm/25 mm		
31		
Long-term therapy/small veins and chemotherapy		
Yellow/lime		
24		
0.4 mm/21 mm		
24		
Paediatrics/small veins		

Sources/bibliography: 1. Gaukroger PB, Roberts JG, Manners TA. (1988). 2. McKee J, Shell J, Warren T, Campbell V. (1989). 3. Van Carrapiett D. (2002). Cannulation Tutorial - Cannula Size [Online] Available: http://www.emergency-nurse.com/resource/iv/iv/size.htm. Cannula Design: http://www.ivteam.com/periphcan.htm

Common abbreviations

A&O	alert and oriented
AAO	awake, alert, oriented
Abdo	abdominal
ABG	arterial blood gas
ABX	antibiotics
ADL	activities of daily living
AKA	above the knee amputation
ARDS	acute respiratory distress syndrome
BKA	below the knee amputation
BP	blood pressure
BPM	beats per minute
CAT	computerized axial tomography scan
CCU	coronary care unit
CNS	central nervous system
CPR	cardiopulmonary resuscitation
CSF	cerebrospinal fluid
CVA	cerebrovascular accident
CVS	cardiovascular system
CXR	chest x-ray
DNR	do not resuscitate
DOB	date of birth
DVT	deep-vein thrombosis
Dx	diagnosis
ECG	electrocardiogram
EEG	electroencephalogram
ENT	ears, nose and throat
ET	endotracheal
FU	follow-up
Hb	haemoglobin
HBP	high blood pressure

Common abbreviations

HR	heart rate
HTN	hypertension
ICH	intracranial haemorrhage
ICP	intracranial pressure
ICU	intensive care unit
JVP	jugular venous pressure
LOC	loss of consciousness
LVF	left ventricular failure
MI	myocardial infarction
MRI	magnetic resonance imaging
N	nausea
N/A	not applicable
NAD	no abnormality discovered
NEURO	neurological
NG	nasogastric
NKA	no known allergies
NKDA	no known drug allergies
Nocte	at night
N/V	nausea and vomiting
ORIF	open reduction and internal fixation
O2 Sat	oxygen saturation
OT	occupational therapy
P	pulse
PH	past history
PMH	previous medical history
post-op	after surgery
pre-op	before surgery
prep	preparations (for surgery)
prn	pro re nata (as required)

Common abbreviations

PTT	partial thromboplastin time
PVD	peripheral vascular disease
R	respiration
RR	respiratory rate
S&S	signs and symptoms
SOB	shortness of breath
stat	statim (immediately)
SURG	surgery
SW	social worker
T	temperature
TPR	temperature, pulse, respiration
Trach	tracheostomy
U/A	urinalysis
URI	upper respiratory tract infection
UTI	urinary tract infection
V	vomiting
VS	vital signs
WBC	white blood cells